REAL
LOVER

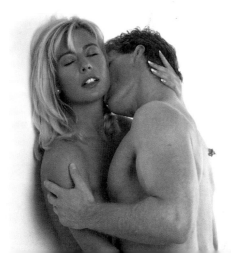

REAL LOVER

BY GRUB SMITH

HarperCollins*Publishers*

HarperCollins*Publishers*
77–85 Fulham Palace Road,
Hammersmith, London W6 8JB

Published by HarperCollins*Publishers* 1999

9 8 7 6 5 4 3 2 1

Copyright © Grub Smith 1999

The Author asserts the moral right to be
identified as the author of this work.

A catalogue record for this book is
available from the British Library

ISBN 0 00 711120 7

Set in Garamond and Futura

Design by design principals

Printed and bound in Great Britain by
Scotprint Ltd. Musselburgh

CONTENTS

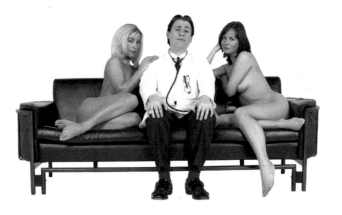

INTRODUCTION

One of the most shameful things about earning a living as a 'sex expert' is that blonde, curvaceous, attractive teenage women always assume I'm going to be great in bed. As a single man, I naturally do nothing to shatter these illusions, but the truth is I'm pretty mediocre. If the act of sex were to be marked by an international panel of judges, a bit like ice skating, then I can assure you I'd be picking up my fair share of 0.5s. The good news, however, is that I am a lot better at it now than I used to be in my twenties, when — like many young guys — I was a dunce under the duvet.

The turning point came when I was dumped by a girl I really loved. Bad sex wasn't the only factor in our split up, but it was an important one. Realising this in the broken-hearted months that followed — months of sobbing and self-pity, of 1½-litre wine bottles and Willie Nelson records — I decided to bone up on the subject. Never again would my foreplay technique rely on a quick nipple tweak and five minutes of lapping away like a thirsty labrador.

During the years that I've been writing the sex column in *FHM* magazine, I've come to suspect

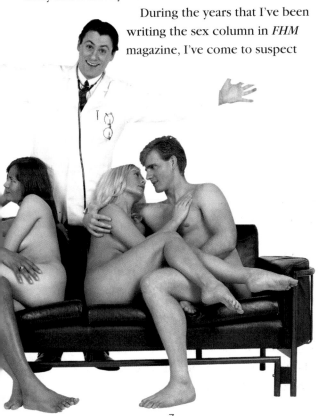

that I'm not the only man looking for answers. I get tons of mail from guys who want genuinely useful details about how to solve their sexual anxieties, rather than the usual flannel to do with 'talking about it' that is commonly dispensed by experts on mid-morning TV shows. That's why I'm writing this book, and maybe it's why you're reading it. It's for anyone who wants to understand how to be better in bed on a purely physical level, and will make you a better, more capable and adventurous lover.

CHAPTER 1
sex drive

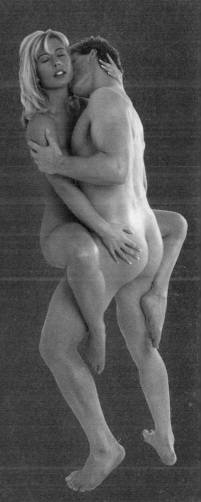

E ven though I possess the most engaging of prose styles, I realise that you spent at least ten seconds looking at that naked woman before beginning this paragraph. And I don't blame you. I would have done too. Because, as men, we have an imperative to check out all the attractive females we see, making mental notes of their good points and wondering if they might go to bed with us. We can't help it. In fact, we even do it when we're supposed to be concentrating on other, supposedly more important matters, as evidenced by this valuable nugget of data:

Number of men who had car crashes when they drove past those Wonderbra posters featuring Eva Herzigova:	**27**
Number of women who had car crashes when they drove past those Wonderbra posters featuring Eva Herzigova:	**0**

But have you ever wondered why we are made this way? Questioned what useful purpose is served by us being slaves to our libido? Mused upon the fact that even rocket scientists and presidents can be reduced to drooling morons with the decision-making powers of a watermelon if their secretary so much as bends down to fasten her shoe? Well, if you have, then I've got some bad news for you: you're reading the wrong book. All that concerns me is that sex is fun. And discovering new ways to make it even more so.

I'm confident, too, that most men share the same sense of priorities. In fact, the most common enquiry I hear is refreshingly straightforward: 'How Can I Make Myself More Attractive to Women?'

The answer? Well, it varies. For every woman who is impressed by the fact that you drive a convertible and know what kind of cheese to buy, they'll be another who thinks you're an insufferable jerk. And the same thing holds true for having large muscles, smoking

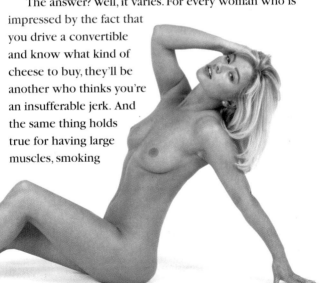

joints, wearing designer togs, enjoying fine art, or cultivating enough chest hair to carpet a small apartment. People have different tastes and what it boils down to is this: sure, Brad Pitt is popular, but even Hitler had a girlfriend.

Nevertheless, having spoken to literally tens of women on this subject, I have highlighted a crucial selection of the things that are definitely *not* appealing to the fairer sex. They are:

● **Cheesy chat-up lines:** Face it, girls are onto these. They've heard them all a hundred times. So when you approach a young lady with your so-called witty opener, she's already biting back a yawn of recognition.

● **Talking about yourself:** Naturally, she wants to know something about you, but on a first meeting this should be kept to a bare minimum. A polite 'What do you do, then?' does not mean she will die unless she immediately hears your entire family history, a detailed monologue about the transmission problems of every car you've ever owned, and numerous ill-disguised lies about how much you earn and how many famous people you know.

● **Preening yourself:** When I was growing up, the

range of grooming products men had to choose from was minuscule. It is generally considered a good thing that we have smartened ourselves up a bit since then. But one unanimous beef among my panel of young women was that men are now going too far in the opposite direction.

● **Not knowing when you're beaten:** If a woman simply doesn't fancy you, no amount of flowers, poetry or Belgian chocolates is going to win her over. Your best bet is to take it like a man, and hope she stays friendly enough to introduce you to her (possibly just as cute) friends. Ah, but how do you know that she isn't just playing hard to get? Well, again, there seems to be a rule here: if you phone her three times in a week and she doesn't call you back, you've got no chance.

So, is there anything positive men can do? Well, a cursory glance at women's magazines (which very considerately appear to run exactly the same features every month, just in case you missed them before) shows that girls are mostly turned on by stuff like 'a sense of humour', 'a kind personality' and 'nice hands'. This may be true, but it isn't very helpful. But, if you read these pages diligently, *Real Lover* may help.

CHAPTER 2
preliminaries

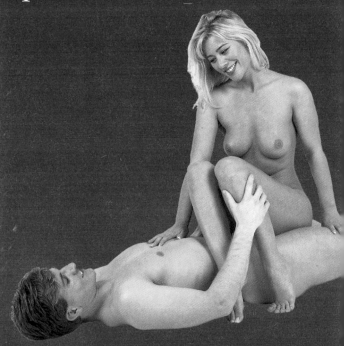

KNOW YOUR BODY

Men, except for the lucky few who earn their living by appearing in such masterpieces of garage cinema as *Raiders of the Lost Arse*, worry far more about the size of their cock than its internal workings. In fact, if personal experience is anything to go by, they worry more about the size of their cock than *anything*, and that includes such comparatively footling issues as nuclear war or global warming.

The normal size of an erection falls anywhere between 13cm and 18cm, depending which survey you believe. If you're unlucky enough to measure less than 7cm when hard, then you have what is called — in a remarkably insensitive piece of medical terminology — a 'micropenis'. And the bad news doesn't stop there, I'm afraid. You see all penises, whatever their size, contain roughly the same amount of nerve endings in the glans at the top. If yours is small, then they'll be concentrated over a smaller area, making you more likely to suffer from over-excitement and premature ejaculation.

8 inches plus: Well over average. Great to show off in the showers after football (and also a handy bookmark for a literary work of this size), but bear in mind that if your partner is 'small', you're going to have to be very slow and careful in positions like doggy and cowgirl.

7 inches: OK, this is no circus cock, but it's the size that women most commonly describe as 'perfect'. However, don't get too relaxed about it — an equally common female gripe is that men who know they are well hung are lazy when it comes to foreplay.

6 inches: Average. You're unlikely to get any complaints, except from the most ardent of 'size queens'.

4½ inches: Frankly, nothing to write home about. But if you study the sections on 'great foreplay' and 'the best sexual positions for men with a small penis', then your abilities and enthusiasm should keep your partner happy.

2½ inches or less: Only about 2% of the adult population have penises this small, so you have a pretty stark choice: either live with it and find a woman who is mature enough not to mind, or consider surgical techniques to enlarge it.

Much ribald humour, but sadly little genuine research, has been devoted to the idea that certain races are better hung than others. For the record, current estimates of the anthropometry of penis size suggest that:

● Men of Asian origin have penises that are, on average, about 2cm shorter than those of their white counterparts.

● Men of African origin can boast an advantage of about 3cm over whites.

● The country which has the largest average cock size is Senegal.

● The Dutch have the longest penises in Europe.

● The Czechs have the fattest penises in Europe.

Although almost certain to finish well ahead of the dog in any list of Man's Best Friends, the penis can cause problems for its owner. Before the advent of feminism, these could simply be ignored or blamed on the woman, but in the vibrant exciting times we live in it's up to us guys to sort these wrinkles out for ourselves. Here are some handy tips.

● **Coming too soon:** A 'hairtrigger' is the most

common sexual complaint that men suffer from. It's usually caused by over-eagerness or anxiety, and though it generally fades with age and experience, it can develop into a serious mental block.

To find out how you rate, you first need to know what a 'normal' length of time to last is. Well, the obvious answer would be 'long enough to make sure you and your partner are both satisfied', and if you assume that the average timespan for a woman to come during sex is about twenty minutes, then that's what you should be aiming for. (Interestingly enough, however, a bed-manufacturing company once did some research on the springing of their mattresses which involved strapping a 'thrustometer' — basically, a jogger's pedometer held in place by a garter — to the thighs of love-making couples. The average number of thrusts in a sex session was only 93.)

If you come up short in this department, then you might consider any of these techniques:

Stopping and starting. When you feel that you are nearing the point of no return, pull out of her vagina and pause for a few seconds until the urgency has receded. You can even turn this to mutual advantage by using the time to give her stimulation with your mouth or hand, or manoeuvring each other into a new position.

Change your thrust. Rather than just going in and out, try leaving your cock deep within her and moving your hips in a figure-of-eight pattern instead. This will provide pleasant friction for her as you grind your body against her pubic area, but leave your sensitive glans relatively unstimulated.

Stick to the missionary. As you are more in control of the thrusting in this position, you will be better able to dictate the pace and slow things down when necessary.

Think about bad things. An old chestnut, yes, but nevertheless some people have achieved good results by doing complex mathematical problems in their heads while shagging. If you're no good at algebra, another popular version is to imagine that your girlfriend is shouting, 'Yes, O Mighty Life Giver, make me big with child.' The thought of a four-year stretch changing nappies certainly works wonders for me, anyway.

● **Not coming for ages:** Although this would seem to be an advantage, especially as it gives the woman more time to climax, it can be a real problem for some men as they get older. Stress and tiredness are common causes, and the condition can also be exacerbated if you're taking anti-depressants or certain anti-histamine drugs prescribed for colds and sinus problems. Alcohol and cocaine can also slow down the time it takes to come, so lay off these before sex if it's a worry.

● **Not getting it up:** A failure to get wood happens to us all at one time or another. Clearly, one reason for it is that you simply don't fancy your partner at that particular time, but it can also be because you fancy her too much. This sounds insane, but I speak from personal experience. Luckily, good old male lust is pretty much certain to override this sort of sensitivity before long, and once you've broken your duck, it should disappear entirely.

As if having a penis to play with at night wasn't proof enough of God's bounty, He has also seen fit to equip us with several other 'pleasure centres'. You will doubtless discover these in the normal course of love-making, but just in case you've been playing things very straight, here are some highlights to watch out for:

● **The G-spot:** Situated just a couple of inches inside your rectum is your prostate gland which, when properly handled, can intensify your climax.

● **The nipples:** Some men can't feel anything in 'em; some can. Don't be afraid to experiment with different pressures and textures, as objects as various as feathers and sandpaper will provide intense stimulation.

● **The perineum:** Not to be ignored by the accomplished fellatrix, when this is lightly caressed it can send thrilling ripples through the whole of the 'downtown business district'. If she can also gently squeeze and 'juggle' the balls while doing this, so much the better.

● **The toes:** It isn't only Fergie who likes having her toes sucked, as you'll discover if you let your babe give you a foot job. The action is the same as if she was sucking you off, and it's best if she reaches forward and masturbates you at the same time. Clearly, if her enjoyment of this act is at all important to you, you should cut your toenails first. And get all the dirt out of them with a penknife too.

KNOW HER BODY

No matter how baffling our behaviour may be to the ladies, at least we men can proudly boast that our genitals are right out there in the open and easy to see. This is not so with women: their sex organs seem to have been hidden with the ingenuity of Anne Frank, contain parts that have to be handled with the dexterity usually reserved for the manufacture of Swiss watches, and — final proof, surely, that God has a crappy sense of humour — are disguised by a thick bush of pubic hair. It is, quite literally, a jungle in there.

Of course, with the possible exception of Mrs Slocombe in Are You Being Served?, *there is more to pleasuring a woman than stroking her pussy. In fact her whole body is a minefield of erogenous zones, and you've got to know how to set off the right explosions. Here, just in case you haven't noticed, are the main areas of interest:*

● **The neck:** Not just a handy target for when Henry VIII wanted to avoid all that bothersome paperwork with the Child Support Agency, it's also the number one place to get a woman's motor revving. Kisses here, if ticklish and feathery enough, will send shivers straight down her spine. But keep it light: she doesn't want to feel your slobber dribbling down her collar.

● **The ears:** Another delicacy, but one you have to treat with respect, as it will definitely not turn her on if you start snarfing on her lugholes like they were Quavers. Instead, try ultra-light nibbling on the lobe (so long as she's not wearing earrings) and the outer edge, alternating this with soft, hot breaths over the whole area. If you've got a nice pointy tongue like that bloke out of Kiss, you can even dart it gently in and out of the hole.

● **The breasts:** Needless to say, touching her breasts will be very exciting for you as well as for her, so there's no excuse for not paying them maximum attention. The golden rule is to start softly as the last thing she wants is some guy attacking her lallies as though they were a dangerous judo opponent. So, begin by caressing the 'valley' between them, then gently cup them in your hands. As you progress, build up the pressure of your squeeze until she lets you know what's perfect. A dab of oil will help things run along even more smoothly and sexily, and you should take care to give both of them equal attention. Crazy as

—

it seems, many women attribute 'personalities' to their boobs, and they may each need different treatment.

● **The nipples:** Once you have fondled her breasts, move on to the nipples. Try circling your fingers around the breasts until they zero in on the areola (the browny-pink bit around the nipple), then gently strumming them. You can also squeeze them or softly flick them between finger and thumb, but avoid any prodding or 'radio tuning' moves, as she'll feel like a piece of unreliable hi-fi equipment. Using your mouth, try blowing on them, then sucking them into your mouth, letting your lips and tongue wet them. Keep your teeth out of things — unless she tells you she prefers 'rough' stimulation — and imagine that you're giving her breast a mini blow job. Above all, just because you're sucking one nipple, don't forget to use your hand on the other one.

● **The back:** Massage is a bore, and in my opinion best left to the Swedes and Turks, but if you can manage to put in five minutes or so of back rubbing, it'll really help to relax your lover. Use a bit of scented oil or baby lotion, slam on some soothing music, and alternate soft stroking with finger kneading. You don't need to know anything about pressure points or physiotherapy — just be gentle and try not to say, 'I've been doing this for ages, are you horny yet?'

● **The thighs:** Stroking and kissing the thighs and the back of the knees before touching her pussy will pay dividends. Your best bet is to skirt around her pubic area, getting closer and closer, but then teasingly pulling away until she's howling for it.

Talking about sex

If you and your girlfriend both want to get the most enjoyment possible out of sex, then it's vital that you're able to communicate your desires. But, even though you both see each other naked a lot, this can be embarrassing. Face it, you probably feel iffy about criticising her technique, because you know how badly you'd be pissed off if she complained about all your hard work under the counterpane. The key note to strike is one of encouragement rather than criticism. Explain to her that what she does is just great, but that it would be even better if she tried such-and-such. Continue the learning process when you're making love. Again, keep a sense of fun about it, giggling if she gets it wrong rather than going 'No! No! No! How many times do I have to show you, woman?'

It might seem premature to be discussing her orgasm at this stage, especially as — in sexual terms — we've barely covered the mechanics of getting her coat off, but I figure there's no harm in being aware of what you're aiming for. And a woman's orgasm is a far more complex thing than the eager, easy jolt you and I enjoy so much.

For a start, while men can have orgasms pretty much at will, hers will require more than merely supplying the correct physical stimulation. She'll almost certainly have to be in a receptive frame of mind as well. (And, though I know I promised not to bombard you with statistics, the laboratory research figures show that fewer than 1 in 10 women can be made to 'trigger' an orgasm involuntarily.) The physical side of things, however, goes like this:

Women can have two kinds of orgasm. The first, and most common, is the clitoral orgasm, brought on — as the name cunningly suggests — by direct stimulation of her clitoris. This will happen mostly through foreplay; only in very few sexual positions is the clitoris angled correctly to get rubbed against the shaft of your thrusting cock.

Her climax will follow certain set stages: arousal, when she gets wet and her labia fill with blood; plateau, where her sensations of pleasure flatten out before the climb to orgasm; orgasm itself, which lasts about ten seconds, and in which her vagina will be subject to spasms and muscular contractions; and post-climax, where she'll slowly float down from the ceiling again. Once she's come, she probably won't want to be touched, as her clitoris will be incredibly sensitive.

The second kind of orgasm is the vaginal one, which only about 20 per cent of women claim to have. Caused by the sensations she feels inside her pussy, and probably directly linked to G-spot stimulation, it's less dramatic and characterised more by a warm glow of contentment throughout the body than any banshee shrieking and bucking about.

CHAPTER 3
foreplay

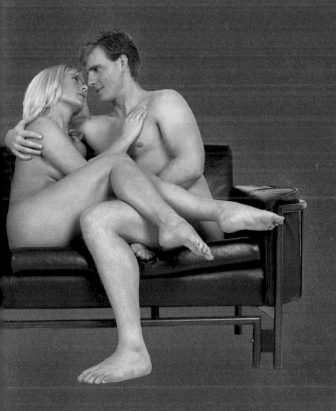

Through sex education, we are now all aware that it takes the average man about three minutes to come, but that the average woman needs twenty minutes. Even more encouragingly, most of us are now clued up to the fact that the solu-tion to this disparity is not to send your girlfriend upstairs with an erotic novel and a long-handled hairbrush, then ask her to give you a shout after seventeen minutes. No, we recognise that there's a job to be done, and that we have to do it.

There is still, mind you, a world of difference between trying to give good foreplay and actually succeeding. So let's kick off this vast section by laying down some ground rules. For a start, there's the word itself: foreplay. This suggests that kissing, stroking, biting and licking are activities that should be attempted only *before* sex, whereas the lover seeking plaudits should be prepared to do them throughout the whole performance, from soup to nuts. And afterwards, too. Bear in mind also that getting into a set routine is lethal to passion, so instead of going through your regular moves each time as though they had been choreo-graphed as rigidly as a minuet, mix things up. Begin foreplay way before you intend to go to bed, teasing her for hours with kisses and caresses, stopping and starting until she is really fired up and raring to set the sheets ablaze. When you're in bed, punctuate each break between positions with cunnilingus or finger-work, and — especially if you have a small cock — try to make sure she comes at least once before you do.

Above all, when you are caressing her breasts and private parts, keep this motto in the forefront of your mind:

'Do everything half as fast and twice as softly as you think you should.'

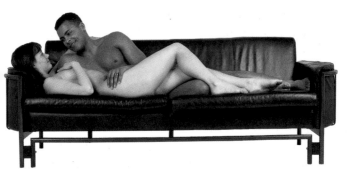

Kissing

An accomplished lover will spend more time on kissing than on any other sexual activity, so you shouldn't just see it as an irritating stop on the way to your ultimate destination. Also, as first impressions count, a good technique could be the difference between going home with a woman and sleeping alone.

Take note that with kissing, as with dining, good manners are everything, and try these methods out for size…

● **Soft kisses:** Keep your lips almost closed at first, and kiss her mouth incredibly softly, switching to cover every millimetre of its surface area, with special attention being paid to the corners. Then, keeping your lips as dry as a cocktail party in Jeddah, move them over the contours of her face, lingering on her neck, collar bones, cheeks and ears.

● **Blowing:** As you are moving your mouth over her face, try blowing — again, with infinite subtlety — on her skin. You'll need to have a Colgate 'ring of confidence' in your breath to stop grossing her out, but if you alternate between cold and warm blows, it can have a tantalising effect.

● **Butterfly kisses:** Why limit your kissing by using only your mouth? In this popular method, you flick your eyelashes across her face. Although tricky to do well, and not necessarily doing that much for her, it may make you seem like the last word in sexual sophistication.

● **Lip chew:** When you begin to kiss with open mouths, it's a good idea to gently lick her lower lip with the tip of your tongue, and then 'suck' it into your mouth. When it's trapped between your teeth, gently bite down and twist it, pulling it slightly away from her. Again, the key word here is gentle. (You can also try this with her upper lip, but it's a lot more difficult. And your noses get in the way.)

● **Gum kisses:** This is no walk in the park to do well, and it's best ignored unless you have one of those nice, pointy tongues. It works like this: when you're kissing, bend your tongue tip upwards and run it across her gums where they meet her front teeth. If you get the pressure right, you will send pleasurable tingles across these nerve-endings, which are the most sensitive in the mouth.

● **Jousting tongues:** With your mouths held slightly apart, let the tips of your tongues flicker over each other's surfaces, changing from a back-and-forth to a figure-of-eight motion, and not ignoring the side of her tongue either.

● **Tongue swapping:** As abandoned as it sounds, so wait until you're both warmed up before giving it a whirl. Basically, you take turns to give each other's tongue a blow-job, taking it into your mouth and sucking and slurping along its entire length. You'll be drawn right up against each other when this happens, so don't forget to supplement it (and all the techniques mentioned above) with…

● **Using your body:** Great kissing is not just about doing the right things with your mouth. Your hands should also be busy, stroking her neck, squeezing her manfully to you, perhaps even caressing her face and hair (although that *really* annoys some girls). If you're lying down at the time, you can also use your feet to massage the sensitive insides of her calves, or just wrap your legs around hers like a python sizing up a plump goat around dinnertime.

Handwork *Turning You On*

If you're serious about making your love life more exciting, then you need to put extra time aside for it. And this time is best employed warming each other up before you actually begin to fuck. While you probably won't want to attempt all the moves listed below in a single session, you can still use just one or two to make each sexual encounter more memorable. First up, the tricks she can perform for you…

● **Double hand job:** This one requires a bit of dexterity and rhythm. With you lying on your back, she kneels between your legs and places her right hand round the base of your cock. Her left grips loosely on your helmet. She brings her right hand up, passing it under the left one and off the top of your cock. Then, as her left hand goes down, she moves her right back to the base, where left passes over it. And so on. This is also a lot easier to do if you're well lubed, and once she gets the hang of it, get her to incorporate a slight twisting motion rather than just sticking to a straight up and down.

● **Corkscrew hand job:** Frankly, some women aren't much cop at handwork, and they seem to have copied their one boring technique from that Nescafé gesture popularised by Gareth Hunt. However — as everyone wants to be good in bed — she probably won't mind getting some tips, so encourage her to test out a variety of simple alternatives. This one involves her using her grip to travel up and down your cock in a corkscrew motion, and it can be made even more pleasurable if she uses a lubricant like baby oil. (Bear in mind, though, that this tastes pretty foul, so you'll need to wipe it clean with a towel if you want her to suck you later.) Her spare hand can be used to play with your balls or G-spot, the techniques for which are listed later in this section.

● **Finger-job:** Instead of simply yanking your foreskin up and down, in this method she uses a slight vibrating motion with one hand around the glans. As an added attraction, she also constantly passes her thumb over the wet surface of the helmet, caressing the sensitive nerve-ends.

● **Downwards hand job:** A variation on the above, this is supposed to feel as though your cock is constantly entering her pussy. Each of her (well-lubricated) hands takes it in turn to pull downwards on your cock, squeezing around the helmet as it does so. Understandably, this one can hurt if she's not gentle, so make sure she knows your limitations. Especially if you're uncircumsised.

● **Scrotum tickle:** While wanking you off, she can use her spare hand to cup your balls. If she also employs her fingertips to tickle forwards, using a very light touch, the effects on the sensitive skin can be highly arousing.

● **The G-spot probe:** As discussed in the 'penis' section earlier in this book (see page 16), correct stimulation of your G-spot can improve an orgasm. So, when you're close to popping your cock, she can slide a well-trimmed — and preferably well-greased — finger an inch or two inside your arse. This is obviously a lot easier if she's positioned near the lower half of your body beforehand.

● **A little bit of 'Spanish':** Why the 'breast wank' should be named after our Andalucian cousins I have no idea, but it is. I don't make the rules up. Anyway, this works best when you're lying side to side and quite close to orgasm, at which point she holds her breasts together, enveloping your penis. You then help out by thrusting away. Clearly, this works best if she has large boobs, and a spot of baby oil won't go amiss either.

Handwork *Turning Her On*

Now it's her turn. Again, bear in mind that no woman will want to experience all these moves in one session, so ration them out until you know which ones are guaranteed to get her smokin', and which ones simply don't hit the right spot. It will really help you to learn how to give her pleasure if she allows you to watch her masturbate, but if she's shy about this there's a useful compromise. When you start to touch her pussy before sex, just keep your finger still and get her to grind and wriggle against it. This will give you a good idea of the target area, and also clue you in to how hard or soft she likes to be caressed. Once again, and in an even bigger type size, I emphasize:

'Do everything half as fast and twice as softly as you think you should.'

● **The warm-up:** After you've treated the rest of her body to foreplay, begin to stroke her thighs, letting your hand trail softly up one and then down the other, pausing only momentarily over the pussy. Then make each stroke shorter, so you're beginning to zone in on her vagina. Let your fingers teasingly caress the really smooth skin of her upper, inner thighs, and then finally run one finger up and down the crease formed by the labia. Don't attempt to penetrate her yet: just glide gently over the outside.

● **Kneading:** Place two fingers along the length of her labia, and use a soft kneading motion to stimulate her. You can move your fingers slowly all the way from the mons pubis to the perineum while doing this. If she's still dry after a few minutes, lick your fingertips and run them on the inside edge of the labia, but — again — don't try to touch her clitoris or get inside her yet.

● **The pubic pull:** Place the heel of your hand on the skin just above her pubes. Lock a few hairs in between your fingers and gently pull them in a swirling motion, taking care to cause pleasure not discomfort. You can simultaneously use your middle fingertip to touch her pussy.

● **Making circles:** When her pussy begins to open up, dip your finger slowly inside to moisten it with the natural glandular lubrication. Then rub this fluid around the clitoral area, avoiding direct contact with the clitoris itself, and instead making small circles

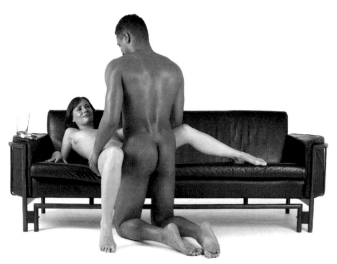

or figures of eight around the base or hood.

● **The pop out:** Using two fingers held closed together, make small, delicate circles over the clitoris. Then place the fingertips on either side of it and press them in towards her body, making clitoris 'pop' out. You can then use your other hand to caress it.

● **Cupping:** Placing your palm over her pubic hair, bend your middle finger so it's angled to touch her clitoris. While applying gentle downward pressure with the heel of your hand, use your finger to rub her clitoris up and down, in circles, or to strum it subtly like a guitar string. If you keep the two fingers next to it straight, they can caress the edges of her labia.

● **Scissors:** Place two fingers all the way inside her pussy, then open and close them like a pair of scissors. You can do this either vertically or horizontally, but make sure's she's very turned on or the stretching feeling may hurt her. As will your fingernails unless they're well manicured.

● **The pistol:** Close the four fingers of one hand into a point, keeping the thumb up at right angles so that the whole thing resembles a cocked pistol. Use the ball of the thumb to stroke her clitoris while you plunge the fingers in and out of her pussy. Try to adopt a twisting motion as well as an in-out one, and, naturally, ensure she's wet enough to take this bantamweight version of 'fisting'.

● **The dipped finger:** Alternate dipping a finger into her wet pussy and slowly sliding it out of her in an upwards direction. As it heads towards her navel, it's entire length will roll against her clitoris, and — if you care to keep up the rhythm of this sawing motion — it's a good way to ensure she comes.

A relaxed woman is less likely to feel nervous or uptight, so the best way to ensure you can bring her off with just your fingers is to tell her she's got all the time in the world. And mean it. And, while it's great to show what a virtuoso you are with different techniques, remember that once she nears the 'home straight', you should stick to a steady rhythm and just one method. Stopping and starting something new is only going to set her back a few minutes. Be aware also that her 'ideal point of pressure' can change from hour to hour, so don't assume that what worked last time will necessarily work again. Lastly, if she's experiencing real trouble in coming, she can help by clenching and unclenching her buttock and vaginal muscles, and sometimes just by pressing the soles of her feet together.

Oral Sex *Blow Jobs*

Forget black and white. Forget Christian or Muslim. In reality, the world is divided into just two types of men: those who love getting blow jobs, and those who are dead. The most remarkable thing about this state of affairs is, of course, that so many women are lousy at giving head. Sure, they'll put their lips around your cock, and they may even bob up and down a bit without making it seem like they're doing you the world's biggest favour, but that's not the same as getting it right.

But you don't have to put up with that any more. If you're prepared to make an effort by learning some of the moves in this book, then so should she. And you could do a lot worse than leave this section open on her bedside table…

● **Preparation:** Clearly, hygiene is incredibly important here. But, as it may surprise you to learn that her mouth is home to far more germs than your old fella, it isn't just a matter of you giving your tackle a once over with Imperial Leather. No, she should also make sure she's had a good brush and floss too. And, as watching her mouth work on your penis is always much more fun that simply viewing the back of her head, you should make sure she's positioned in such a way that gives you panoramic views of the whole business.

● **Basic blow jobs:** If she's nervous about giving head, which usually happens if she thinks she might choke, then get her to keep one hand gripped around the bottom of your shaft, and don't do any thrusting yourself. Once she's happy, she should make an 'O' with her lips, keeping her teeth well away from the action, and simply slide up and down, using her tongue to keep your penis wet. The act of licking saliva onto your shaft for this purpose should naturally provide enough swirling stimulation to make you come. But to make things more sensational, ask her to experiment with…

● **The hand up:** Instead of simply holding one hand around the base of your penis, get her to lift it up and down in rhythm with her mouth. She can either tug it in the opposite direction to her lips — taking care not to stretch your skin too far — or do it in tandem with her lips, thus giving you a simultaneous hand and blow job.

Cunnilingus

A damned ugly word, cunnilingus (from *cunnus*, the vulva, and *lingus*, the tongue) is also a damned difficult thing to do well. For a start, vaginas are tricky things to navigate. When you consider that a clitoris can be as small as a grain of rice, and that it's concealed beneath a jungle of pubic hair and two folds of flesh, it's no surprise that so many men just lap away haphazardly, like a blind man ducking for apples. What makes matters worse is that women rarely offer assistance. Perhaps out of politeness, gratitude, or just plain insecurity about the appearance of their genitals — once memorably categorised by Martin Amis as varying between 'the greasy waistcoat pocket and the slashed vole's stomach' — they are reluctant to bark out the sort of Golden Shot style instructions we'd be happy to hear. Nevertheless, if you try out these tips on your girlfriend, I guarantee she'll soon be dragging you upstairs come bedtime.

● **Preparation:** A lot of men muff-dive for the wrong reason — because it's the quickest way to get their lover wet enough to penetrate. If this is your attitude, change it. For cunnilingus to work best on her, she has to know that a) you love doing it, and b) she's got all the time in the world. (Get her in this state of mind, of course, and she'll actually climax *faster*, because she won't be tense.) So, don't treat it as a chore or a race, make sure you pay proper attention to the rest of foreplay first, and when you do begin to lick her pussy, don't dive straight for the clitoris. The key word is 'lingering'.

Also, as many women worry about the flavour of their vagina, put her at ease with a comment like 'I love the way you taste' or even a simple 'mmmm' of pleasure. Above all, don't ignore the other parts of her body just because you're giving her head, and try not to leave her in the cold by taking all the duvet down there with you. Once you've got these points straight, prepare for any problems you might face, such as…

● **Jaw ache:** Cunnilingus can be a tiring business, and there's a good chance you'll begin to feel cramp in your jaw or tongue. If this happens, try keeping your mouth still and making the movements just with your neck, or get her to grind her pussy against you while you take a break.

● **Stubble:** The George Michael look may go down well with the girls in a club, but on the soft skin of their faces, thighs and pussy it's often less popular. If you rub against her too harshly or for too long, she may get a minor rash that'll be painful for a day or so. If this is a real dilemma, then try softening your bristles before bedtime, either with a shaving balm or normal shampoo.

● **How do I know she likes it?** Trust me, you could get long odds at Ladbroke's on her *not* enjoying oral sex. But if you're worried that she's not getting turned on, try this easy experiment. If her erect clitoris begins to shrink and retract during muff diving, then you're doing something wrong. Either switch to handwork, or ask her how she would prefer you to lick her out.

● **Basic cunnilingus:** This is your bread-and-butter muff-diving, but it's none the less effective for that. Start by kissing her labia majora softly, using only your lips, as though kissing someone hello at a party, and then probe your tongue into her labia minora as she begins to wetten. Move up to the clitoris, but kiss *around* it rather than straight onto it. Use your fingers in any of the ways described earlier in the 'Hand Work' section (see page 35). Lick it gently, using a combination of circular or up-and-down motions, sticking to just one as she approaches climax. It's fine to change the rhythm at the start, but keep it regular once she nears the finishing line (or the chances are she'll never get there). As for the pressure, it's a personal choice, and one you should let her make. If she presses her pussy hard into your face, she probably wants it stronger, and vice versa.

● **Blowing:** Some women respond very well to soft blowing on their pussy and, especially, their clitoris, so long as you do it subtly rather than like someone trying to get a fire going in the wilderness. Be careful, however, to keep your breath on the outside of her: if you actually blow *up* her vagina, it can cause a fatal embolism. And I bet she's going to let you try *this* one now.

● **The 69:** No foreplay technique has achieved quite such a legendary status as the 'soixante-neuf' — which is surprising, as it's not particularly satisfying. Sure it's intimate, sure it's democratic, but it's hard for her to concentrate on coming herself if she's worried about sucking you off, and you yourself are at a poor angle to lick her clitoris. Personally, I think it's wiser to stick to the 'onze' or '11', a position where you lie parallel but take it strictly in turns to pleasure each other.

● **The orgasm suck:** When you sense that she is beginning to come, try sucking her clitoris into your lips and holding it there. This will intensify her feelings of orgasm, but make sure you're ready to release it if she gets too sensitive to be touched after her climax.

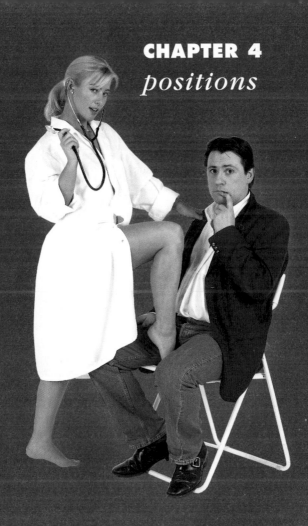

CHAPTER 4
positions

Once you have mastered the art of foreplay, it's time to look at the many different ways there are of making love. Most of us still only use three basic positions when we're making love. Of course, they're great and they do the job, but if you want a long relationship to stay exciting it's best to know some extra moves.

Next we come to the question of when and how to try them out. As many of them require a good deal of forethought, co-ordination and practice to get your limbs in the right position, it's best not to spring them on a girlfriend unawares. Perhaps the best solution is to learn them together beforehand, but even then I would recommend moderation. A change in positions should come naturally, and if you start barking out instructions like 'Number 43! Then two minutes of number 17!' she's going to feel like an over-worked waitress in the Golden Pagoda.

Above all, know your limitations. Although new positions may help you both find a different kind of bliss, and pausing to adopt each new variation will help you delay ejaculation naturally, without having to think about long division problems, they do require a certain level of fitness.

But there are bound to be some new delights for you in the pages which follow. So enjoy ...

MAN ON TOP *positions*

Most people associate this style with boring sex, probably because it was the position officially sanctioned by Victorian missionaries. When these worthies arrived to convert Africa, they were horrified to find that the natives were accustomed to shagging in every posture under the sun, often going so far as to enjoy themselves. Quick to pounce on any activity more pleasurable than singing 'Kum Ba Yah' in the round, they insisted that everyone stick to the so-called 'missionary position', a technique in which the man does press ups while the woman lies underneath him pretending to be dead. Now, liberal commentators might be tempted to speculate, in a smart-arsed *Guardian*-reading way, who were really the 'uncivilised' ones here. But not me. Mainly because the Africans also worshipped raccoons.

However, the point is that man on top positions don't have to be dull. Indeed, they have many good points to recommend them. It's easier to control your rate of thrust (and thus your orgasm) for instance, and it leaves her hands free so she can use them to caress your back or play with your anus. On the minus side, some of them are pretty hard work on the arm muscles, it's difficult to use your fingers to stimulate her clitoris while doing them, and most of them result in relatively shallow penetration. Nevertheless, remember the wisdom of the phrase 'nothing ventured, nothing gained', and give these a crack. Not all of them are startlingly different from each other, but sometimes even the slightest change can add a slice of novelty to your routine…

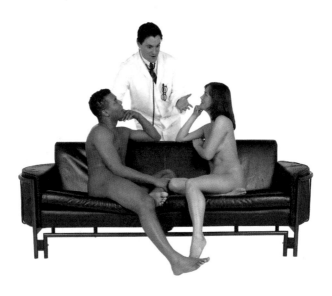

POSITION 1 *The Foot Stroke*

How to do it: She lies on her back underneath you, with her legs quite widely open and her feet hooked between your legs.

Good points: This differs from straight missionary sex because the woman uses her feet to push up and down along your thighs, setting a rhythm and gently scratching you with her toenails. Also, as both your bodies are pretty much constantly pressing against each other, there is excellent skin-to-skin stimulation.

Bad points: Not particularly flattering unless you're both in tip-top physical shape. Your gut will hang down, and her breasts, if not extremely firm, will flop to the side. (Mind you, a good suggestion if she's self-conscious about this, is for her to keep her upper arms pressed into her ribs, as this will perk her breasts up to a near-silicone standard of firmness.)

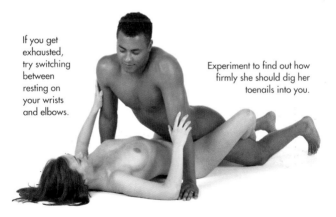

If you get exhausted, try switching between resting on your wrists and elbows.

Experiment to find out how firmly she should dig her toenails into you.

POSITION 2 *Crossed Feet*

How to do it: You keep yourself raised high above her, entering her vagina quite steeply, while she crosses her ankles over your bum or back.

Good points: She can pull you inside her, thus giving her control of the pace and rhythm. Also, because she has her thighs lifted, you will get a better angle for deeper penetration, and be more likely to rub against her clitoris.

Bad points: You have to stay up on your wrists most of the time.

Her legs dictate the desired speed of your thrusts, which is especially arousing as she approaches orgasm.

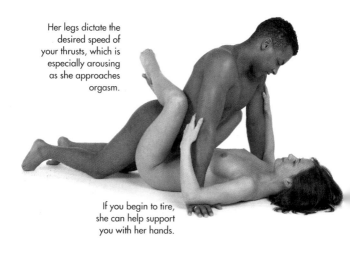

If you begin to tire, she can help support you with her hands.

POSITION 3 *Meeting Halfway*

How to do it: Keeping yourself elevated on hands and knees, you let her lift her pelvis from the bed. You then do 'half thrusts' each in mid-air.

Good points: In this position the woman can buck against you, meeting you stroke for stroke. This gives a nicely abandoned, animal feel to the proceedings. (If you want to see it done well, watch the famous opening bonk scene in the movie *Betty Blue*.)

Bad points: If you have a short penis, you're likely to 'slip out' quite a lot. And if you mistime your thrusts, you could get a painful knock on the end of your old fella.

If she keeps her hands on your arse, there's less chance of you losing the rhythm.

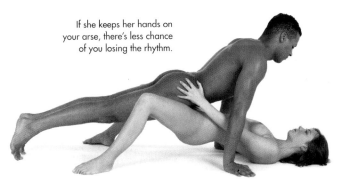

For maximum appeal, keep the rest of your bodies from touching.

POSITION 4 *The L-Shape*

How to do it: You squat back on your calves and, gripping her by the waist or hips, softly pull her body towards you on each stroke.

Good points: Visually very appealing, as your partner is all stretched out below you. It's easy to lean forwards and stroke her breasts or stomach, and similarly to have her suck on your fingers while you screw.

Bad points: Shallow penetration, not much ease of movement, and it's bloody impossible to kiss unless she has the abdominal muscles of a trained gymnast.

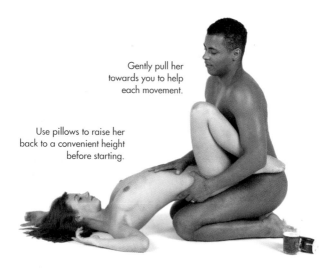

Gently pull her towards you to help each movement.

Use pillows to raise her back to a convenient height before starting.

POSITION 5 *The Press*

How to do it: Simple. Just lie on top of her, and get her to slide her legs over yours so she has some purchase for thrusting.

Good points: Extremely intimate, as your entire bodies — from head to toe — are touching.

Bad points: Shallow penetration. Severely restricted range of movement. And a very real chance you may squash her, so don't even dream about it unless you are a) well hung, and b) tipping the scales well under the light-welterweight limit.

Rub the length of your legs against her soft inner thighs as you rock gently back and forth.

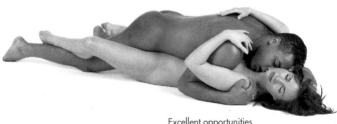

Excellent opportunities for kissing her neck.

POSITION 6 *Grip the Headboard*

How to do it: Go to the top end of the bed and hold yourself in place with your hands. Grip on the sheets with your toes for extra hold.

Good points: Gives you excellent leverage and is less exhausting than most man on top positions. You can even free up one hand for caressing her breasts.

Bad points: Useless if you sleep on a futon.

Good grip allows for
firm, deep penetration.

Her hands are free to stroke
or scratch your back.

POSITION 7 *The Lotus Position*

How to do it: Kneel on all fours above her, and carefully help her cross her legs into the Lotus position. Always make sure she is comfortable, especially when you start to lie some of your weight across her.

Good points: Extremely unusual and inventive, so it's unlikely you'll have done it with too many other women. Gives a slight whiff of bondage, which may be a turn-on for you or your partner.

Bad points: She must be very supple to manage this position, so don't attempt it with anyone who flunked yoga class. Also, as her legs will be pushing your body up and away from her, you need to have a long cock to get anywhere.

She can rock back and forth, but her movements will be more restricted than normal.

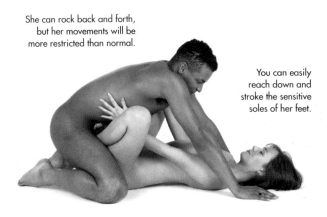

You can easily reach down and stroke the sensitive soles of her feet.

POSITION 8 *Foot on Chest*

How to do it: Like the next three positions, this is a variation in which the woman uses her legs and feet to help you rock back and forth. In this version, you squat back on your calves, and she supports herself by resting one outstretched leg on your thigh. The other leg is bent so that the foot pushes into your chest.

Good points: It's ideal if she gets her jollies from a toe job, as you can administer one while fucking her, instead of just keeping it for foreplay. Plus, the folded pose effectively constricts her vagina, so it's a good option for guys with short penises.

Bad points: She can't do much with her hands, and her knee will inevitably cover one of her breasts. Even if she's thinner than Kate Moss, the bending of her torso may make her feel that she looks fat. Also, it's a bugger to untangle if you suddenly need to answer the phone.

Make sure she's washed her feet. Obviously.

Given the precarious nature of this position, it's best to vary in-and-out thrusts with figures of eight.

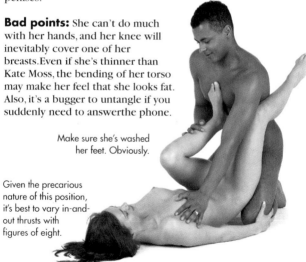

POSITION 9 *The Deckchair*

How to do it: She lies on her back, with both her legs curled back onto her chest. She rests the soles of her feet against your chest, while you bend your body so you are fucking 'downwards'.

Good points: Very deep penetration, so it's perfect for the less well-hung. It's also easy to fondle her arse and to reach between her legs to stimulate her clitoris. Plus, it's worth noting that this position will 'tense' the muscles of her vagina, helping her build up towards orgasm.

Bad points: It's possible to hurt her by thrusting too hard, so you have to go slowly and carefully. It's probably not the best position to finish off in, especially if you get really carried away when you come. Also, a real no-no if you prefer to get your rocks off when looking at her breasts.

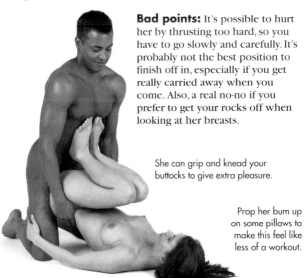

She can grip and knead your buttocks to give extra pleasure.

Prop her bum up on some pillows to make this feel like less of a workout.

POSITION 10 *The Legover*

How to do it: The woman lies slightly on her side, twisting so that her right leg goes over your left shoulder, or vice versa. It's essential to prop her up with pillows so that her pussy is at the right height for penetration.

Good points: Your balls can rub against the soft skin of her thighs as you move in and out, and — visually, at least — you get the best of both worlds, being able to see her tits and arse cheeks.

Bad points: Unless she fancies a trip to the leg fractures ward of your local hospital, it's impossible to kiss her. Plus, penetration will not be deep, especially if you have a gut.

Both hands are free to caress her body.

You can maintain a rhythmic scratching of her thigh in time with each stroke.

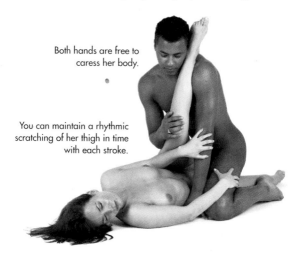

POSITION 11 *The Double Legover*

How to do it: As with number 10, except she puts both her legs over one of your shoulders. Oddly enough, this makes manoeuvring much easier, so you should get a more active romp.

Good points: Very deep penetration. Allows you to stroke the backs of her thighs and calves, and to kiss her feet during the action.

Bad points: Uncomfortable if she's not very lithe or gymnastic. Plus it's almost impossible to stimulate her clitoris like this, so make sure that she's well warmed up beforehand.

If her knees are kept pressed together, this will 'tighten' the vagina, causing extra friction on your cock. And thus more pleasure.

It's easy to change from vaginal to anal sex without any fussing about.

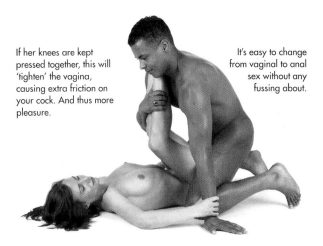

POSITION 12 *The Knees Up*

How to do it: The woman rests her feet on her partner's hips, giving her some purchase to thrust back at him during sex. He arches his back and uses short, shallow thrusts.

Good points: Again, quite a dominant position for the guy, allowing him to push down on her with each thrust. He can easily fondle her breasts and — by opening her knees — lean forward to kiss her. Because of the angle of penetration here, the shaft of your cock should also be able to brush against her clitoris.

Bad points: Not a great deal of scope for moving around. She may object to being folded up like a parcel. And she won't be able to do much with her hands, either.

Lean forwards to tease her nipples during sex.

Keep her steady by squeezing your thighs around her butt.

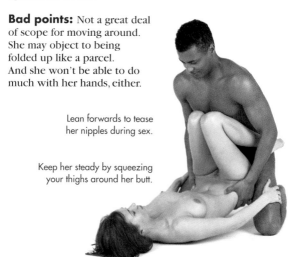

POSITION 13 *The Hand Grip*

How to do it: You kneel forwards and point your erection downwards so that it meets her vagina, supporting yourself by gripping her hands. Be careful not to put too much weight on her, however.

Good points: With her thighs wide open and her legs stretched out behind you, this is an extremely horny, pornographic position. Although penetration isn't particularly deep, it allows you to lean forwards to kiss her mouth, neck and breasts.

Bad points: Very tiring, especially for her. And you can't use your hands.

Raise her arse to the required level by using a cushion or pillow.

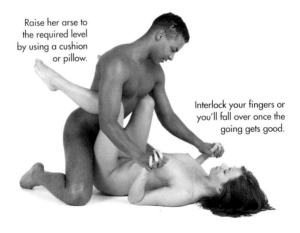

Interlock your fingers or you'll fall over once the going gets good.

POSITION 14 *The Collar*

How to do it: She lies on her back with her hips raised to facilitate entry, and places her feet on your shoulders. You support her weight with your thighs.

Good points: If she keeps her thighs together as much as possible, this position will 'tighten' her vagina. It also provides an excellent angle for deep penetration, and both of you may find the submissive nature of it very arousing. Plus, she can easily reach between her legs to masturbate while you fuck her.

Bad points: You have to do most of the thrusting, although she can help by gripping your legs or forearms.

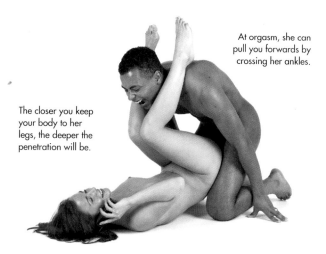

At orgasm, she can pull you forwards by crossing her ankles.

The closer you keep your body to her legs, the deeper the penetration will be.

POSITION 15 *The Open Wide*

How to do it: She lies on her back with her legs pulled up, and you hold them in place with your arms.

Good points: This is one of the best positions for deep penetration, so make sure she's fully turned on before attempting it. It's also one of the most dominant, so you're totally in charge of how hard and how fast you wish to thrust.

Bad points: If you have a big cock, you have to be careful or you could cause your lover pain with this one. It's also tiring on the arms, which have to bear all your weight.

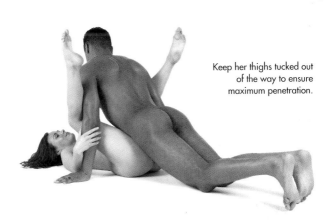

Keep her thighs tucked out of the way to ensure maximum penetration.

POSITION 16 *The Lazy Kneel*

How to do it: She lies back on the bed with her legs over the side, and you kneel in front of her on the floor. Depending on the height of your bed, you may need to use cushions to get the angle right.

Good points: No weight on your arms, so it won't be tiring even if you're not exactly Brian '*Superstars*' Jacks. Very easy to touch her breasts and clitoris while you're at it.

Bad points: You'll be quite far apart from each other, so kissing is out of the question.

She can easily reach down to masturbate herself.

Hold onto her hips to stop her sliding away from you on the 'outstroke'.

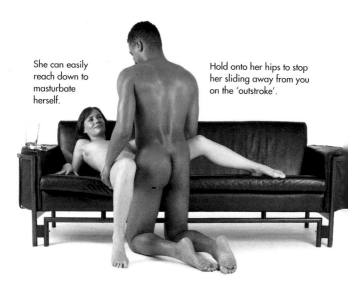

POSITION 17 *The Riding High*

How to do it: You squat astride her, arching your back so your cock is at the right angle to enter her pussy. She can support you by folding her legs behind your arse.

Good points: Excellent for clitoral stimulation because you're coming 'down' on her. As you're holding her thighs together with yours, her pussy will seem tighter than usual.

Bad points: Shallow penetration, so small-cocked guys can expect to slip out quite a lot. Plus, you have to be cautious when thrusting or you might bruise your penis.

You may need to use your hands for balance, so playing with her breasts could be a precarious business.

Use short thrusts to ensure stability.

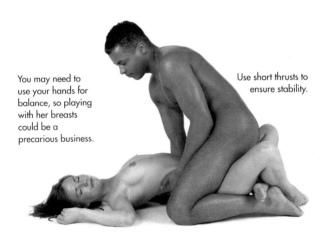

GIRL ON TOP *positions*

The keen-eyed amongst you will have noticed that the positions in the previous section required men to do most of the 'work'. So what better to try next than some techniques in which you lie flat on your back, attempting nothing more athletic than a sickly leer of satisfaction?

Not that your partner will think you're lazy if you guide her into a 'girl on top' (or 'cowgirl') position. On the contrary, she'll probably be delighted, because it'll give her a chance to set the pace and rhythm of sex, to regulate the depth to which your cock penetrates her, and to generally be the dominant one in bed. As well as all this, these positions afford her much more room for manoeuvre than when you're squashing her, so she'll find it easier to reach down and touch her clitoris during sex.

Visually, too, they are a treat. You can usually see your penis sliding in and out of her pussy, and her breasts will be displaying their natural heft instead of disappearing towards her armpits. On the minus side, it'll be harder for you to control your orgasm, so premature ejaculators should be ready to warn their partner when matters are approaching meltdown. You should also make sure that you're good and hard before initiating this kind of shag — a floppy cock is more likely to slip out, and if she brings her weight down on it you could be looking at the sort of groin/pain interface more commonly associated with peasant being asked to sign a confession by the Chilean Rapid Response Police Squad.

One last point before we get onto the dirty pictures. It will really improve your pleasure if your girlfriend is fit enough to squat up on the soles of her feet, rather than simply rest her shins on either side of you. In this position, she can add all manner of delightful twists and figure-of-eight swivels to the proceedings as she rises and falls. So, just as she may be using her subtle feminine wiles to encourage you to lose weight from your gut, you could do worse than tell her to use the step machine next time she's at the gym.

POSITION 18 *The Jockey*

How to do it: You lie down as though out sparko, and she sits on her haunches (and your penis). She may need to put her hands on your chest for balance, and you can use yours to stroke her thighs or breasts.

Good points: If she opens her legs, you'll be treated to some very horny views of her riding your cock. This is an ideal position for her to show off her virtuosity in the saddle. Also, it offers excellent penetration.

Bad points: Tiring for her. You can't really do much thrusting, so you may feel a mite submissive.

You can reach up to cup and play with her breasts.

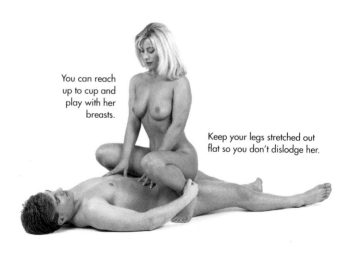

Keep your legs stretched out flat so you don't dislodge her.

POSITION 19 *The Lazy Jockey*

How to do it: As the name suggests, this is a less vigorous version of the previous style, mainly because she can rest on her lower legs and sit back on your thighs.

Good points: It's easier to fondle her tits like this, and — providing you're not a complete slob — you can easily sit up and kiss them too. She has both hands free to pleasure you (or herself) with.

Bad points: Penetration, though still impressive, isn't quite so deep as in 'The Jockey', and she'll find it harder to do any gymnastic trickery.

Put your thumb against her clitoris to provide stimulation as she rides you.

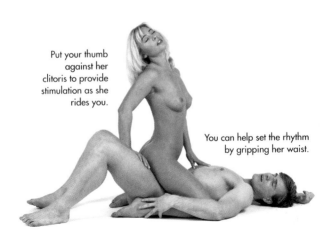

You can help set the rhythm by gripping her waist.

POSITION 20 *Backwards Cowgirl*

How to do it: You lie on your back with your knees apart and slightly raised. She sits between them facing the other way.

Good points: All the advantages of doggy style, but without the carpet burns, this allows you to massage her back and buttocks while you fuck. You can easily finger her anus, and she can reach down to fondle your balls. Best of all, she can lean forwards until she finds the perfect angle for G-spot stimulation.

Bad points: Can feel a bit impersonal if you get your jollies from eye contact. And it's a law that you have to keep saying how nice and small her arse looks.

Reach up to caress her spine or pull on her hair.

The faceless aspect of this position makes it ideal if you want to fantasise about making love to someone else.

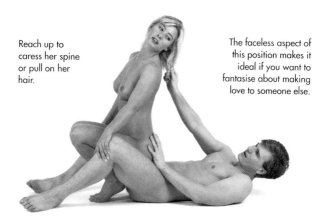

POSITION 21 *The Nice Lie Down*

How to do it: Yup, you're flat on your back again, but this time you have to take her weight because she stretches out on top of you, getting as much skin to skin contact as possible.

Good points: She can rotate her hips to give very different sensations to the usual in-out-in-out ones. If she's a tall girl, you can kiss deeply while you fuck.

Bad points: Because she doesn't support herself on her elbows, she could squash the breath out of you if she's been packing away the cakes recently. And the slowness of this style makes it a bit 'Sunday morning' for more athletic tastes.

Her movements should be slow
and subtle, rotating and grinding
rather than rising and falling.

She can rest her feet on
yours to give added
purchase.

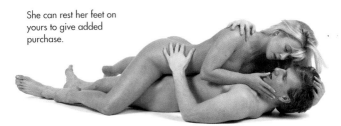

POSITION 22 *Criss-Cross*

How to do it: Sit up with your legs outstretched while she sits facing you. Lean back and grip each other by the ankles. Let her do the rocking back and forth.

Good points: It's different, and it has a nice element of mutual bondage as you're holding each other in place. Superb views of her pussy writhing on your cock.

Bad points: A bit unwieldy, and penetration is quite shallow. Also it bloody hurts your ankles if she puts too much weight on them.

Kissing is impossible, so make the best use of eye contact to turn each other on.

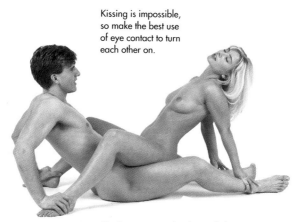

Don't try to tug on her legs to help the rhythm — it won't work.

POSITION 23 *The Interlocking Position*

How to do it: She wraps her legs over your arms while sitting between your legs. You hold her in position by resting your hands on her back.

Good points: She can lean forwards to kiss you. You can toy with her nipples. And you feel a bit of a stud, frankly, for even knowing this position exists outside of a game of 'Twister'.

Bad points: No picnic to get into, and once you're there penetration is nothing to write home about. Movement is also fairly restricted.

If she rests back on her hands, it frees yours up to caress her.

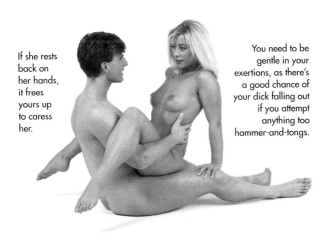

You need to be gentle in your exertions, as there's a good chance of your dick falling out if you attempt anything too hammer-and-tongs.

POSITION 24 *Rising to the Trot*

How to do it: You sit upright and she goes astride you, crossing her legs and holding onto your back for support.

Good points: She can only really generate any bouncing motion by squeezing her thighs up and down, so for many women this position is reminiscent of horse-riding. As this action will cause her vaginal muscles to contract, you should feel subtle waves of pleasure as though your penis was being 'milked'. It's also a great one for touching and kissing her tits.

Bad points: The gentle rocking motion may be a little tame for some tastes. And if you're a fat bloke, she won't be able to get close to your cock.

Ideal for kissing her neck and breasts.

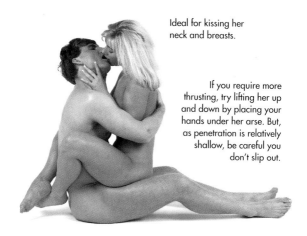

If you require more thrusting, try lifting her up and down by placing your hands under her arse. But, as penetration is relatively shallow, be careful you don't slip out.

POSITION 25 *The Crucifix*

How to do it: Once again, you're out flat on your back like one of the boy Tyson's opponents, except this time you have your arms outstretched. She climbs aboard, linking hands with you, and you mutually flex your arm muscles to help her rise and fall.

Good points: Excellent for kissing while your fuck, and if she's quite light you can get a surprising amount of movement going. You may also get turned on by the faux bondage element here.

Bad points: Definitely a bit too subtle for some tastes, and she'll need to have good control of her vaginal muscles or you're not really going to get anywhere. Also, if she's a bit of a porker, you could end up going blue in a hurry.

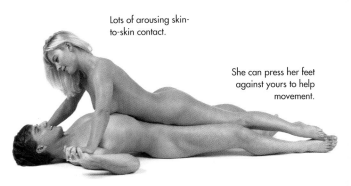

Lots of arousing skin-to-skin contact.

She can press her feet against yours to help movement.

POSITION 26 *Crossed Legs*

How to do it: She sits in a loose lotus position on top of you, resting one hand (and as much of her weight as possible) back on your knees. You support her by holding her up with your thighs and hands.

Good points: If you're knackered, then this allows her to masturbate and to be totally in charge of things. She can rub your erection over her vaginal lips and clitoris in between strokes, and she can angle it so that her G-spot is stimulated. All you have to do is watch.

Bad points: Her crossed legs mean you can't actually see that much action. And if she's lardy, you could end up feeling that you've been run over by a bus.

You can lick your fingers and reach up to her nipples while she bobs away.

If your cock is long and flexible enough, she can lean back to get different sensations in her pussy.

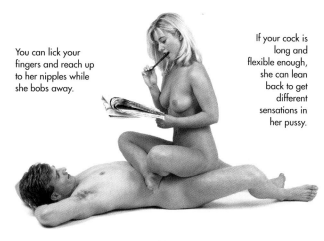

POSITION 27 *The Seesaw*

How to do it: You sit up with your legs extended and quite wide apart, holding her with your hands so she can lean backwards. She grips your arms and lowers herself onto your cock.

Good points: Easy to lavish attention on her breasts with your mouth.

Bad points: It's pretty hard to thrust in this position, and you can only use one hand on her tits or she'll be in danger of falling backwards. The angle of penetration isn't particularly comfortable if you've got major wood

Use one hand
to caress her
neck, spine
and hair.

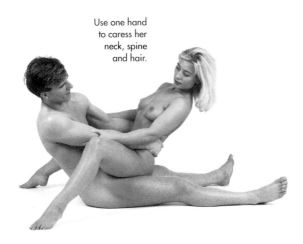

POSITION 28 *Lying Back*

How to do it: You're sitting with your legs open wide enough for her to lie in between them. Once you've pulled her onto your erection (which will have to be held down to facilitate entry), you can hold her knees together to 'tighten' her vagina. She rests up on her elbows.

Good points: You're very close to the action if you pop your cork by watching her pussy doing the old sword swallowing act. Unlike most other 'girl on top' positions, you can dictate the pace by pulling her thighs back and forth. Also, the angle of your cock is certain to stimulate her G-spot.

Bad points: You really have to bend your cock down to get it in. She can't use her hands to any productive purpose.

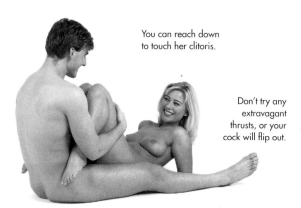

You can reach down to touch her clitoris.

Don't try any extravagant thrusts, or your cock will flip out.

POSITION 29 *The Wraparound*

How to do it: This is pretty much a human knot, so I wouldn't recommend it on a first date. What you do is sit with your legs crossed and get her to lower herself onto you, bracing herself on your thighs and curling her legs around your ribs.

Good points: Both of you can set the rhythm by lifting and pushing against each other. You're close enough in to be able to bite or kiss each other's necks, lips and shoulders.

Bad points: Frankly, a bit uncomfortable for both parties, so don't even think about it if you've got backache. Plus, she can't touch your balls and you can't reach her pussy, so it's only worth a crack if she gets off on vaginal sex.

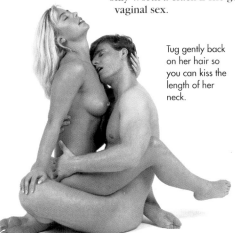

Tug gently back on her hair so you can kiss the length of her neck.

She can push off your knees to get 'lift'.

POSITION 30 *Leaning Back*

How to do it: She wraps her legs around your back, leaning her weight back and supporting herself by grasping your ankles. Your hands are free to caress her back, armpits or breasts.

Good points: If she's light enough to be manhandled, you can jog her up and down on your erection. You have both hands free to explore her body. It's easy to lean forwards and kiss.

Bad points: Neither of you can touch her clitoris, and this position won't work too well if you've got a beer gut.

Ask her to move her hands every now and then, or your shins will start to ache.

If her legs are short, she won't be able to cross them behind you.

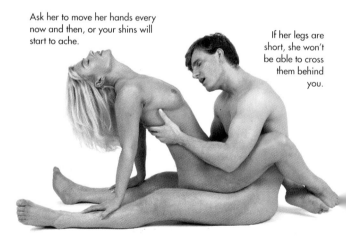

REAR ENTRY *positions*

It is a matter of no small mystery to me how something as pleasurable as rear entry sex ever got the nickname 'doggy style'. Because anyone who has ever watched dogs fuck will be able to tell you that they have absolutely *no* style at all. I mean, we're talking about an animal whose idea of foreplay consists of drooling, and which will gladly hump furniture or your trouser leg if it can't find a slow enough bitch to rape in the local park.

Similarly, when people talk about rear-entry sex being good because 'it brings out an animal instinct', I begin to wonder if they've ever seen any of those nature programmes on TV. Because, whether David Attenborough happens to be pointing his camera at bugs, baboons or birds, one thing is immediately clear — they sure don't look as though they're enjoying it much. The females, especially, can forget any human refinements like cunnilingus or the multiple orgasm: a good fuck for them is one where they don't actually fall out of the tree afterwards. In short, whoever it was who wrote that 'Nature is red in tooth and claw' might just as easily have added 'and it sure as hell doesn't own too many Barry White records either.'

With regards to the human race, however, rear-entry sex is one of the very finest ways available for achieving mutual ecstasy. Penetration is nearly always extremely deep, the penis is angled to chafe agreeably on the G-spot, and — because there's no eye contact — both partners have free rein to fantasise about making love to a mystery partner. As well as this, her breasts will be more sensitive because gravity will increase the bloodflow to the nipples, and your scrotum will brush against the soft cushion of her buttocks with each stroke. OK, on the down side, it's easy for anyone with a hairtrigger to lose it in this position, precisely because it's such a visual and sensual feast, but — hey! — look on the bright side. What other position allows you both to pull utterly abandoned 'come faces' without worrying that you look like a Romanesque gargoyle?

POSITION 31 *The... oh, alright then... Doggy Style*

How to do it: She gets down on all fours as though searching for a lost contact lens, and you plug yourself in from behind. Easy.

Good points: She's going to feel plenty of even the smallest cock in this position. During sex, she can reach back and touch her clitoris or your balls, and you can lean over to cup her breasts. Plus, if you get the timing right, you can both do the thrusting.

Bad points: Both your knees may suffer from carpet burn, and short-legged fellows may need to prop themselves up with cushions or switch to the Rifleman (see position 33).

If you're fat, you can rest your belly on 'nature's shelf' — her arse.

By sliding a finger down the crevice of her butt cheeks, you can stimulate her anus while you screw.

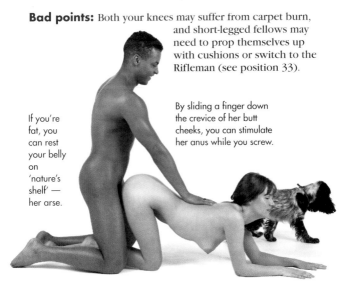

POSITION 32 *Passive Rear Entry*

How to do it: It's essential that you use a soft bed for this one, as the floor — even if lushly carpeted — will be too hard for her. Once you're on top of the duvet, she lies down with her legs parted enough for you to fit in between them. Ride away in the press-ups pose, taking care not to collapse on top of her.

Good points: Very submissive for her. Presuming she likes that sort of thing.

Bad points: Penetration is pretty shallow for a rear-entry position, the view is terrible, and neither of you can do anything useful with your hands.

Arch your lower back to get extra penetration.

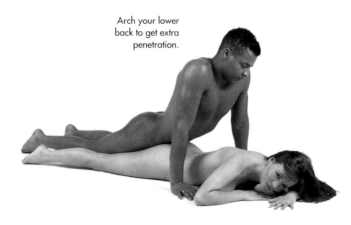

POSITION 33 *The Rifleman*

How to do it: As with Doggy Style, she's on all fours and you're stationed behind her. However, you go up on one knee, which will raise the height of your tackle about 3 inches. This could be crucial if you're a bit shorter than her.

Good points: All the advantages of doggy, but with the added bonus that it stops you clambering all over her like a climbing frame.

Bad points: None whatsoever.

Don't try to go up on both your haunches — you'll look like a goblin taking a dump.

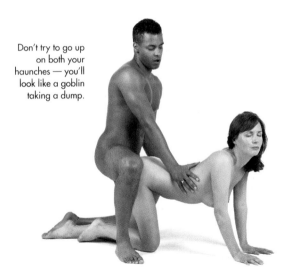

POSITION 34 *Riding Backwards*

How to do it: You lean back on your arms, she squats on you and leans forwards on hers.

Good points: She does all the humping, and can angle your penis inside her for maximum satisfaction. If your legs are open wide enough, she can reach back to caress your balls.

Bad points: You're a bit inactive, and it can be a strain on the back and arms. She's laughing, mind you.

Once she has come, she can up the ante for you by squatting on her soles intead of her shins. This will provide a real show and guarantee deeper thrusts.

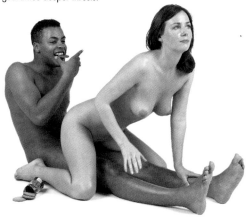

POSITION 35 *Standing Doggy*

How to do it: She bows down facing away from you, resting her palms on the floor to add stability. You grip her waist and do your bad thing.

Good points: Top notch penetration, extremely dominant, and you can control the depth of each thrust.

Bad points: As her head is pointing down, blood will flow there, possibly making her feel a bit dizzy and short of breath. So this one is only really suited to a quickie fuck in which you want to be the boss.

Try not to tug her back and forth too much, as it's hard enough for her to maintain balance already.

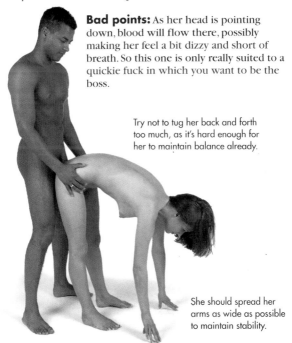

She should spread her arms as wide as possible to maintain stability.

POSITION 36 *Reverse Cowgirl*

How to do it: You lean back and she sits slightly sideways on top of you, with one leg passing over yours, and one underneath. She provides all the motion necessary by rising and falling on her thighs.

Good points: You can kiss her neck, and she can use her two free hands to rub her clitoris and your balls simultaneously.

Bad points: You're pretty much the passenger in this one, so it would be a bit of a damp squib if you feel particularly randy and active.

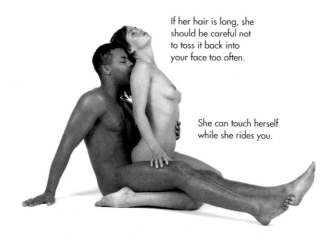

If her hair is long, she should be careful not to toss it back into your face too often.

She can touch herself while she rides you.

SIDE-BY-SIDE *positions*

Very much the poor relation of the three main sexual
styles, side-by-side positions (and I'm including here,
for the sake of argument, standing-up sex) are
nevertheless worth trying, especially if your erotic life
is getting jaded. They offer plenty of body contact and
hands-free action, there's no danger of being crushed
by a fat partner, and they are ideal for comfort if your
lover is up the duff. Best of all, standing-up sex is
superb for dangerous or outdoor quickies, whether
they're up against a tree, in a shop changing room, or
35,000 feet high in the luxurious surrounds of an
aircraft khazi.

The only real problems crop up if you and your
partner are noticeably different in height, in which case
the knee-bending and back-arching necessary to hit the
bullseye make them more trouble than they're worth.

It's also relevant here that one of the most popular
and intimate sexual positions falls into the 'side by side'
category. Known to most people as 'spoons' — but,
bizarrely, to men in the Armed Forces as 'a lazy sailor' —
it's almost unique amongst sexual positions because
neither partner has to do any work. And, just as Marilyn
Monroe once remarked that 'ageing, powerful men

seem to prefer me on my hands and knees', so it might be pointed out that 'knackered couples who feel horny but don't want to miss out on watching *Friends* while having sex prefer doing it on the sofa like spoons. I mean, so they can watch the TV at the same time.'

Although, admittedly, that's less catchy.

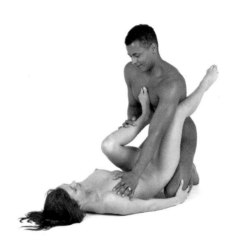

POSITION 37 *Sideways On*

How to do it: Piece of cake — you lie full length next to each other, she raises her top leg so you can slip your old fella in, then you put your leg on top of hers to 'close the door' again.

Good points: Once you are holding her top leg down with yours, her pussy will be tight as a drum, guaranteeing great friction for you and — given the proximity of your groins — lots of stimulation for her as well. You can also do a lot of cuddling and hugging in this position, which the ladies love, eh?

Bad points: Penetration isn't amazing, and the whole event may be a little too gentle for some tastes.

Her entire genital area will be pressed against yours, ensuring plenty of sensation.

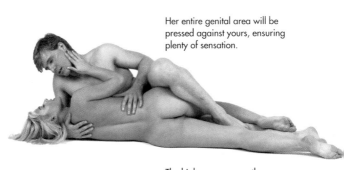

The higher up you go, the more the shaft of your cock will rub against her clitoris.

POSITION 38 *Stand Up*

How to do it: Supporting one of her legs with your arm, you bend at the knee until you're able to get your cock inside her. Brace the leg she is wrapped around so she can use it to help her thrust back at you. It's also a good idea to do this up against a wall rather than free-standing.

Good points: Lots of kissing and stroking of arse, breasts and back. And having a quickie is always fun and liberated because she's probably not expecting to get an orgasm out of it.

Bad points: A bit unwieldy. And a disaster if she's taller than you. I mean, you'd need a trampoline to get anywhere.

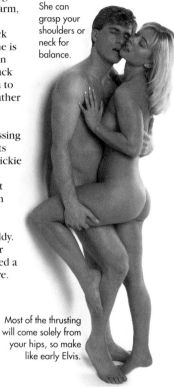

She can grasp your shoulders or neck for balance.

Most of the thrusting will come solely from your hips, so make like early Elvis.

POSITION 39 *The Scissors*

How to do it: So called because it looks in profile like a pair of scissors, this position is really only viable for the guy who's packing a large cock. She guides you inside her then places both her legs over yours.

Good points: You get to feel her arse a lot. And, of course, her breasts and lips are ready and waiting.

Bad points: Anything under 6 inches just isn't going to be in far enough to light the blue touchpaper, I'm afraid.

Pull her down onto your cock with each thrust or you may slip out.

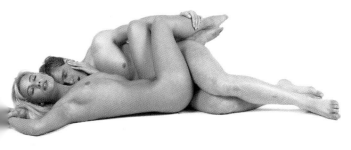

POSITION 40 *Spoons*

How to do it: Ideal for making love on a sofa if you're both watching TV, this is one of the simplest and least strenuous positions to pull off. Just lie behind her on your side, raise her top leg until you can slide your cock home, then gently thrust in and out.

Good points: You're entirely skin-to-skin, and you can hug or caress every part of her. Kissing the sensitive nape of her neck couldn't be easier.

Bad points: You won't be able to French kiss without one of you ending up in a neck brace. She can't really do much to you with her hands.

Hold onto her hip to
keep things stable.

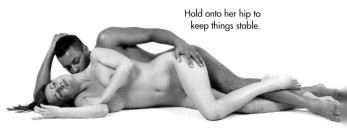

Reach round to touch her clitoris or
breasts while you fuck.

POSITION 41 *The Grab*

How to do it: You lean back against the wall, and your girlfriend grips her hands around your neck. You then help to pull her up, holding onto her thighs or arse for support. She gets what foothold she can on the wall behind you, and the fun begins. Alternatively, you can swap over so she's against the wall.

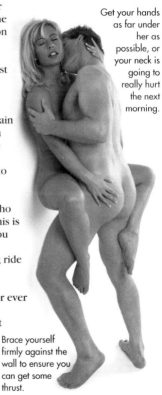

Get your hands as far under her as possible, or your neck is going to really hurt the next morning.

Good points: Ideal for a quickie in a cupboard or a train khazi, and it could give you a kick just to know that you're strong enough — and your girlfriend is slim enough — to manage this.

Bad points: For anyone who hasn't been pumping iron, this is a real trial. And, given that you can't really get a lot of movement, it's frankly a long ride for a short slide. On a more practical note, there's also a chance that your wall will for ever bear the marks of your girlfriend's dirty toes. So best save this one for when you're staying in a hotel, eh?

Brace yourself firmly against the wall to ensure you can get some thrust.

POSITION 42 *The Entwined Position*

How to do it: You lie parallel to each other, with your lower legs stretched out straight. Your top legs cross over, with hers wrapping around your butt.

Good points: Great for kissing and stroking each other's bodies, and she can set the tempo by pulling you in with her foot. Penetration is actually pretty good for a side-by-side style, but as her pussy is 'open', it won't feel so tight around a little fella.

Bad points: This is a very 'loving' position, as opposed to one suited to primeval and abandoned banging, so there isn't much action. Also, while you can use your fingers to stimulate her arse, she has no chance of returning the favour.

As you're so close together, there's no chance of clitoral stimulation. So stick to caressing her arse.

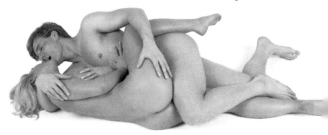

Wrap your foot around her calf to get extra grip.

POSITION 43 *Standing Behind*

How to do it: She braces herself against the wall, with her feet apart. You bend down to enter her, then stand up, lifting her off the ground if necessary.

Good points: At last, a position that's superb for small guys, as the less you have to lift her, the easier it's going to be. That said, it's not really as comfortable as standard doggy, and its main attraction seems to be that you can kiss her neck while screwing.

Bad points: Another one that's going to do your magnolia walls no favours, I'm afraid. And it's very submissive for the woman, so don't expect her to do anything fancy with her hands. Unless she's double-jointed.

The wider apart her feet are, the easier it will be for you to gain entry.

COMPLEX *positions*

Although they failed to come up with the concept of
'the sandwich' until well into the eighteenth century,
our ancestors nevertheless proved themselves to be
highly inventive creatures. Nowhere is this ingenuity of
mind so clearly demonstrated than in the number of
ways they devised to make love. In fact, you might be
surprised to learn that — from the Romans to the
Mayans to the Samurai — they conceived of over 500
different sexual positions.

However, I've picked just seven 'complex' ones for
this book, because I honestly believe that no one likes
having to constantly rearrange their body parts during
sex. And frankly, even these seven should be saved until
your love life gets really, really boring and you've tried
all the other normal stuff, because they are neither
comfortable nor easy to carry off. In short, try these on a
first date and your new lover is probably going to think
you just got out of jail. After serving a very long sentence
for a very weird crime.

That's not to say there aren't any good things about
them, of course. For starters, they are probably a lot
'dirtier' than most of the stuff you and your partner have
done before, and — whatever your parents, your teachers

and your priest may have told you — sometimes it's nice to be filthy. Also, to be a truly open and adventurous lover, you can't afford to turn your nose up at new ideas, however strange they may seem. Your motto has to be 'try anything once'.

So, if you're in good shape, it's a special occasion, and your girlfriend gives you the green light, you could do worse than check these out and get weaving.

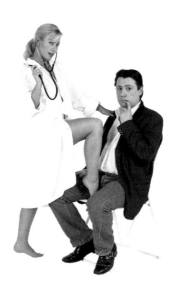

POSITION 44 *The Turn*

How to do it: You lie back while she rides you, cowgirl style. Then, using her hands to steady herself, she lifts one leg over your body and begins to turn sideways. She carries on rotating, stopping at each point of the compass for a few thrusts until she's gone full circle.

Good points: You get a unique corkscrew feeling on your cock while she turns around, and — like one of those 'multiple' postcards from a holiday resort — you get a full view of all the goodies she's got.

Bad points: She needs to be very nimble and very wet to manage this. And it's best to hold onto her in case she slips, doing you a very nasty injury in the process.

Keep still and let her do the majority of thrusting, or else it'll feel like a rodeo for her.

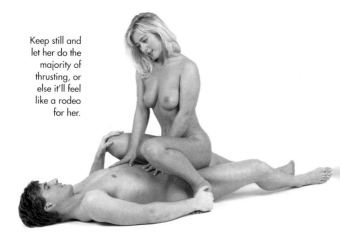

POSITION 45 *The Slide*

How to do it: Jesus, this isn't easy, but if you're determined to have a crack, then kneel down and lift your girlfriend's legs up to your shoulders. Next, holding your erection downwards, slide it into her. Anyone packing less than seven inches need not apply.

Good points: Well, it's probably more fun than cribbage. But only just.

Bad points: For you? Well, bending your cock like this won't be terrifically comfy, but you've still got by far the easier draw here. As well as strain on her lower back and creases in her stomach, she's soon going to find the blood rushing to her head. In short, for show-offs only.

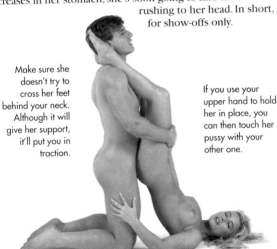

Make sure she doesn't try to cross her feet behind your neck. Although it will give her support, it'll put you in traction.

If you use your upper hand to hold her in place, you can then touch her pussy with your other one.

POSITION 46 *The Wishbone*

How to do it: Slightly more tricky to arrange than 'a quiet night in' with Oliver Reed, this is one sexual position that you'll actually have to choreograph beforehand. She starts by lying across the bed, with one leg raised, then you slide in behind her at right angles. Next, bend your legs forwards so she can hold your ankles, then grip onto her shoulders to provide purchase for your thrusts.

Good points: Another one for your collection of novelties. Plus, she can give your feet a good rub down…

Bad points: Apart from the palaver involved in getting into this shape, you'll probably find that it makes her lower leg go numb after a few minutes.

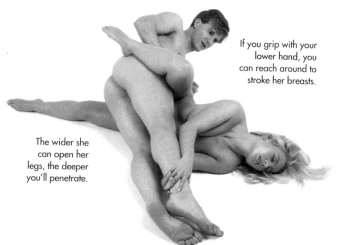

If you grip with your lower hand, you can reach around to stroke her breasts.

The wider she can open her legs, the deeper you'll penetrate.

POSITION 47 *The Missionary Turn*

How to do it: Similar to 'The Turn' except that *you* have to be the one fit enough to appear on *Gladiators*. The trick is to keep as much weight off her as possible, and to slowly swivel your body around in a circle without letting your cock slip out.

Good points: Gives you a chance to explore every part of her body, from head to toes. The different angles of penetration will also afford both of you a full range of sensations.

Bad points: Bloody exhausting on the arms, and at one point you need to bend your cock backwards — no picnic if you've got major wood. Plus, it's pretty essential that she keeps quite still during the proceedings, and at one stage she also has to look right at your arse crack. And, well, it's not Venice, is it?

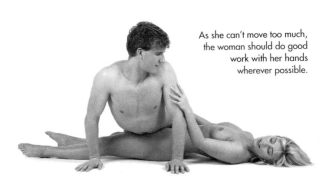

As she can't move too much, the woman should do good work with her hands wherever possible.

POSITION 48 *The Toilet Seat*

How to do it: Romantically named it may not be, but this one is worth trying if you want to give her a new sensation. You lie on your back with your knees drawn up, as though preparing to do that odd 'bicycling in the air' routine gym teachers used to be so keen on. She squats down on your penis and lifts herself up and down to provide the action.

Good points: If her breasts are nice, then they will jiggle about appealingly in any handily-placed mirrors as she bobs away. And if you have 'submission' fantasies, then this will really put gravy on your goose.

Bad points: Your cock feels a bit squashed between your thighs, and once again it has to be bent back. Touching each other is well-nigh impossible if you want to keep your balance. And you need to be fit to last more than a few seconds.

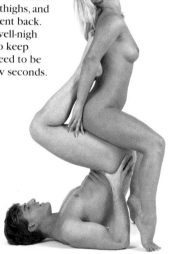

She can hold onto your knees for balance as she rides you.

If you get tired, she can turn 180°, allowing you to lean both your backs against a wall.

POSITION 49 *The Fold Up*

How to do it: You make like a four-legged creature, and she lies underneath, pulling back on her ankles until her pussy is raised up to meet your groin. A cushion or two under her lower back will help matters immensely.

Good points: Fantastically deep penetration, ensuring that even the cruelly ill-equipped will feel like they could audition for *Boogie Nights*. Also, it's reassuringly filthy.

Bad points: You can't caress her, and she's so busy holding her legs in place that she won't be able to do much either. She'll need to have signed up for a few stretching exercises too.

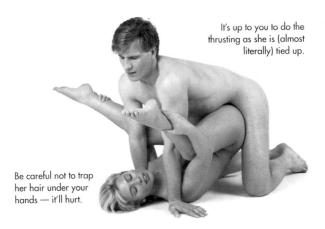

It's up to you to do the thrusting as she is (almost literally) tied up.

Be careful not to trap her hair under your hands — it'll hurt.

POSITION 50 *The Wheelbarrow*

How to do it: Stand behind her, then lift her up by her thighs, pulling her back onto your cock while she supports herself on her hands. It's actually possible to walk around the room while doing this one, but she might appreciate it more if you just stick to thrusting.

Good points: So long as she's not too heavy, you can get some good in-out motion going here. And if laughing is as much a part of your love life as it should be, then you're sure to get some fun out of this.

Bad points: Neither of you can use your hands for anything exciting, and she may get a rush of blood to the bonce.

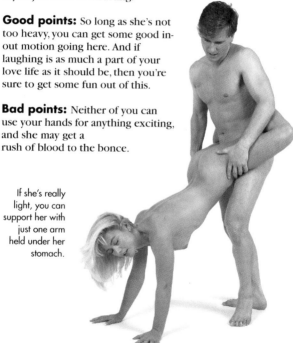

If she's really light, you can support her with just one arm held under her stomach.

A SHORT WORD AT THE END...

I sincerely hope that *Real Lover* helps you to enjoy your love life more. When freed from its attendant anxieties, sex has a wonderful, unifying power that can strengthen the bond of love; it's free; it's good exercise; and it sends people off to work in a good mood, thus resulting in a cheerful, industrious population and a boost to productivity.

So read this book again, and get under that duvet. The recession ends here.

Guy Smith.

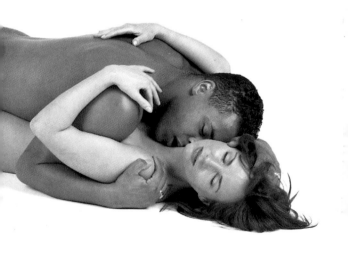